Also by Dr. Stenbeck

Available from the usual on-line source

Books

Healing Yourself -- The Holistic Approach
  [An introduction to Holistic Self-healing.]

Heal Yourself Right Now!
  *[The Seven Priority Organ Levels for
  effective Nutritional/Holistic Treatment of
  all organs.]*

**The 22 Unique Body Types
  (for Health and Weight Loss)**
Q & A to Identify Your Body Type (Booklet)
  [Individual Type booklets are also available

Booklets
  (Step-by-step instructions on healing yourself)

#1 Start Healing with Positive Thinking
#2 Mastering Positive Feelings for Health!
#3 Spiritual Balance and Your Healing

The Eldic Body Type

The Dustin Hoffman, Hillary Clinton Celebrity Body Type

For Kaye,
there at the beginning with Doc Severn,
and for Liberty,
continuing the holistic healing journey...

Disclaimer

The information in this book is for educational purposes only and is not a substitute for medication, diets, or other medical care. The diets do not treat diseases or medical conditions, and are an adjunct to your orthodox health care.

The author and publisher accept no responsibility for any misuse of the information within. If you have any physical problem, food allergy, emotional disorder, or disease, common sense dictates that you consult with a physician before changing your diet, taking nutritional supplements, or following the advice given here.

About the Author

Educated in New Zealand and in the U.S.A., Dr. Stenbeck attained B.Sc. (NZ), M.S., and D.C. degrees. His holistic healing methods have been profiled in magazines (Esquire, McLean's, Playgirl, the Atlanta Constitution), and on TV in the USA and in Canada. He was the main contributor to the Warner Book, _The Eye/Body Connection_ by Jessica Maxwell that focused on the holistic healing relationships between the iris structure and organ genetics.

In the 1970-80's he was elected Fellow, Royal Society of Health, London; Fellow, American Association of Chemists; Member, American Association of Clinical Chemists; and Affiliate, Royal Society of Medicine, London. He studied naturopathy and Body Types with Dr. Bernard Jensen and Dr. Clifford Severn, and has practiced in medical partnerships where patients received the joint benefits of medical and holistic healing.

He is a member of Self-Realization Fellowship. To receive advice on any health issue from a holistic viewpoint, or to receive help with your body type, see his web site: *DrStenbeck.net*

———

Contents

* * *

* * *

<u>The 22 Body Types:</u>
Celebrity Examples

This Booklet contains the Eldic type.
[See <u>The 22 Unique Body Types</u> for all type descriptions.]

Thin Types

Atrophic	*Woody Allen / Audrey Hepburn* *Stan Laurel / Calista Flockheart*
Exesthesic	*Cher / Sarah Jessica Parker* *(Female type only)*
Marasmic	*President Obama / Princess Diana* *James Stewart / Kate Blanchard*
Neurogenic	*J.K. Simmons / Joan Rivers* *Jon Cryer / Marin Hinle*
Pathoferic	*(No celebrity males)* *Blythe Danner / Gwyneth Paltrow*
Sillevitic	*David Bowie / Shirley MacLaine* *Rod Stewart / Carol Channing*

Muscle Types

Calciferic	*Michael Jordan / Angelica Huston* *Abraham Lincoln / Grace Jones*
Carbogenic	*George Clooney / Lady Gaga* *Pres. G. Bush, Jr. / Meg Ryan*
Desmogenic	*Marlon Brando / Loni Anderson* *Daniel Craig / Tina Turner*
Eldic	*Ross Perot / Hillary Clinton* *Peter Falk / Sigourney Weaver*
Medeic	*Gary Oldman / Madonna* *John Hurt / Marlene Deitrich*
Myogenic	*Pres. Bill Clinton / Sharon Stone* *Pres. John Kennedy / Julia Roberts*
Nervimotive	*Frank Sinatra / Elizabeth Taylor* *Mark Wahlberg / Natalie Wood*
Nitropheric	*Ben Affleck / Ava Gardner* *Kirk Douglas / Kate Winslet*
Pallinomic	*Pres. Donald Trump /* *Attorney General Janet Reno* *Bill O'Reilly (Fox) / Jane Russell*

Fat Types

Barotic
Robin Williams / "Mrs. Doubtfire"
Elton John / William Conrad

Carboferic
Bill Murray / Roseanne
Billy Gardell / Melissa McCarthy

Hydripheric
John Goodman / Shelly Winters
Wayne Knight / Jennifer Holliday

Isogenic
Einstein / Oprah Winfrey
Phillip S .Hoffman / Queen Victoria

Lipopheric
Rush Limbaugh / Rosie O'Donnell
Chris Christie / Camryn Manheim

Oxypheric
Winston Churchill / Orsen Welles
Ella Fitzgerald / Gerry Spence

Pargenic
Burt Reynolds / Katey Segal
Ron Perlman / Kirstey Alley

Succinct Quote on Human Types

From Victor Rocine, who first described discrete body types around 1900.

"A type is an order of people that differentiates and distinguishes itself by a general and similar form, brain-formation, chemistry, structure, build, immunity, tendencies, predisposition, resemblance, skin-pigment, and type characteristics based on observation and analogy.

"Or, in other words, people of a given type are similar physically and like-minded as if they were brothers and sisters—that is what type means.

"Everything in nature is made according to plan. Man only discovers that plan and gives it a name. The zoologist has not made the animals—he has only described the plan adopted by the wonderful Creator, and named the classes, subclasses, etc.

"How important type research will be to humanity, time alone will make known."

———

Prologue

The esteemed scientist J. J. Berzelius, discoverer of several chemical elements, inspired Victor Rocine to research body types and to investigate the correlation between types and their diseases. Around 1890-1910, Rocine privately published his original findings on the mineral basis of different body types, and this present book exists because of his brilliant insights.

For many years, I studied with Dr. Clifford Severn who had been a personal student of Victor Rocine on body types, naturopathy, herbology, iris analysis, diet, and nutritional healing methods. He had a successful career as a lecturer and healer, and was one of those rare athletes with complete muscle control over his body. I saw him under a spotlight at 85 years of age, contracting and rippling every individual muscle in his perfectly developed body. Field-Marshal Jan Smuts, the WWII South African Prime Minister, devoted a full chapter of his autobiography to how Severn's healing methods had saved his life. In the 1950's, *Life* magazine did a four-page spread on Severn and his family. Fame he had.

Another Rocine student I studied with, Dr. Bernard Jensen wrote of Rocine's body type research and nutritional methods in his privately published book *The Chemistry of Man*.

This book is deeply rooted in Rocine's original work, and with that of Herbert Shelton, M.D., Ph.D. (at Harvard University in the 1930's). I integrated their research with newer dietary and nervous system data along with celebrity examples of each type, hopefully, making this material easier to digest and more entertaining for the reader.

Gayelord Hauser, another Rocine student I knew, was a celebrated health book author. He wrote a popular book on Rocine's types in the 1940's, *Types and Temperaments;* reputedly, he also introduced yogurt to the western world.

This book exists because of Rocine's creative brilliance and original discoveries in natural healing.

▶ *Rocine: "The soul creates the body type."*

Rocine taught that the soul chooses a body type and brain to live in, thus presenting different experiences and life lessons to master. Why were *you* born the way you are?

That is something to think about, especially if it is true! What would your soul purpose be to live in a particular body type. I provide some thoughts on this issue in each type description and try to assess from my experience with your type the particular lessons of life presented therein.

Rocine was as brilliant in his way as an Abraham Lincoln, Michael Jordan, Michael Phelps, Tony Robbins, or a Daniel Day Lewis —all *calciferics*—rare, leaders, brilliant, innovative, and highly intelligent in their different fields of endeavor.

Celebrity examples exist for most types, not a duplicate of you, but someone who has your essence in their body-mind individuality. Knowing your type allows you to become a better you!

The celebrity examples provide further help in identifying your body type.

▶ *Rocine's classic findings are the backbone of this book. Integrated with Sheldon's research and with other dietary and food issues including mental, emotional, and spiritual attributes,*

Many people take nutritional supplements and try different diets without a doctor's advice. If this is your choice, use common sense, listen to body responses, and discontinue any allergic reactions to foods or nutritional substances.

———

The Eldic Body Type

Representing one of the 22 Body Types first described by Victor Rocine around 1900

***

"You may also have a physical or psychological feature not representative of your type such as height, weight, appearance, talent, weakness, strength, etc., due to biochemical errors, environmental influences, racial or cultural differences, and congenital or genetic issues. Nevertheless, the type identification of the average person is usually clear."

— *Victor Rocine*

The Eldic Type: Celebrity Examples

*If you think this is your type, be sure to look at **on-line photographs** of these examples. Look for general similarities to yourself. Note that sub-types cause the differences in appearance between members of the same type.*

NOTABLES

Mother Teresa
Nancy Reagan

POLITICS

President Harry Truman
Presidential Candidate Hillary Clinton
Presidential Candidate H. Ross Perot

Senator Marco Rubio
Prime Ministers Shamir and Yitzhak Rabin
(Israel)

ACTORS

Dustin Hoffman   William H. Macy
Frederick March   George Burns

Jimmy Durante   Burgess Meredith
Hugh Crone
Peter Falk ("Columbo")
Stanley Holloway (Lisa's father in "My Fair
 Lady" movie)

Sigourney Weaver   Christine Lahti
Mary Steenburgen   Sara Miles
Nancy Walker   Sara J. Parker

TV/RADIO

Wolf Blitzer (CNN)   Harry Reasoner
Ed Sullivan   Jack Benny
Katie Couric   Dr. Ruth

VOCAL

Willy Nelson
Loretta Lynn (and many country singers)
Van Morrison

SPORTS

Tracy Austin (tennis)
Tanya Harding (skating)

HISTORICAL

Lawrence of Arabia

OTHER

Truman Capote	Patty Hearst
Artur Rubinstein	Jack LaLayne
Gloria Steinem	
Helen Gurley Brown ("Cosmopolitan")	

[Note: I knew or met three of the above examples, and many others in everyday life, which contributed to my understanding of the type.]

You already know something about this type from their public persona and appearance whether from seeing them yourself or from the celebrity examples. Blend such insights with the type descriptions and the types of your family and friends to discern their presence in your midst!

Read through the types, and if still confused, you may choose to use the personal request for type identification from my web site: *DrStenbeck.net*

———

Eldic Type Questionnaire

These questions describe the generic type, and not specifically you! If any question ever applied to you, then choose the True answer!

For *Question 1 only:*

A = True	B = Maybe	C = Untrue
15 points	7 points	1 point

1. Physically identify with celebrity   ____

Then...

A = True	B = Maybe	C = Untrue
5 points	3 points	1 point

---

2. Height is close to:
   Males: 5'0-5'7   Females: 4'8-5'6   ____
3. Usual weight is close to:
   Males: 120-170   Females: 100-160 ____
4. Body lean or medium-sized; often handsome or attractive; shapely body ____
5. Muscles moderate-sized, strong; may be very strong (Jack LaLayne) ____
6. Are honest, ethical, principled ____
7. Skin freckles are common (like the *desmogenic*) ____
8. High moral sense ____
9. Face has prominent cheek-bones ____

10. Hair dark, red-brown, strong, lovely if healthy; many redheads; maintain full head of hair throughout life; most females like their hair cut short _____
11. Skin tight, strong, tans easily; often have fine wrinkles or cracks on aging _____
12. Invariably kind, friendly, cheerful, likable, optimistic, positive _____
13. Moderate-high athletic ability; able to build endurance strength into old age _____
14. Weight-lift easily (or know are strong) _____
15. Ears notably larger in males; female ears often average-sized _____
16. Lower lip thin, taunt, flat (males) _____
17. Head medium-sized, proportional; higher crown _____
18. Strongly idealistic to help planet, ecology, mankind _____
19. Excellent ability to socialize, converse _____
20. Have distinctive voice; acting, singing, teaching ability _____
21. Intensely patriotic _____
22. Very reliable and dependable _____
23. Courageous: weigh options and act _____
24. Neutral expression and countenance _____
25. Philosophical, peaceful _____
26. Self-activating and entrepreneurial _____
27. Enjoy debate and discussion _____
28. Strong sense of vanity _____
29. When in charge, set rigid rules _____
30. Expect others to live up to your ideals _____
31. Attracted to antiquity, history _____

32. Stand up to be counted on issues _____
33 Blood pressure or heart history
    (or is in the family) _____
34. High self-confidence, image is usual _____
35. Dislike overly-familiarity _____
36. Difficult being diplomats (outspoken) _____
37. 'Thin skinned' if ethics or ideals are
    questioned _____
38. Non-addictive personality _____
39. Often attracted to vegetarianism _____
40. Smile, talk easily; sociable yet distant _____
41. Strong white teeth (yellow with aging) _____
42. Able to inspire and motivate others _____
43. Always happy to help anyone in need _____
44. Slight fat tendency; may gain extra
    10-20 pounds _____
45. Males tough, wiry; females tom-boys
    (tend to dislike wearing skirts) _____
46. Low-set eyebrows; eyes sunken _____
47. Often triangular lower face _____
48. Highly developed sense of loyalty _____
49. Lower lip tight, less-so in females;
    mouth average-size (wider in males) _____
50. Strong chest, full and wide; male has
    light hair; bust comes in all sizes _____
51. High lung volume and endurance _____
52. Back and shoulders strong, muscular _____
53. Abdomen normal-size; narrow hips _____
54. Limbs flexible with strong joints _____
55. Able to take charge _____
56. Reliability and loyalty are key beliefs _____
57. Admire heroic people _____

58. Defend honor, beliefs, and promises   _____
59. Accepting of life events and stresses   _____
60. Have a good sense of humor   _____
61. Talented and often succeed   _____
62. Mind own business (and expect others to do the same)   _____
63. Will not abuse a friendship (are loyal, and expect loyalty)   _____
64. Variable sex drive and sensuality: strong or weak   _____
65. Cannot tolerate injustice or tyranny   _____
66. Are born philosophers   _____
67. Will speak the truth, and fear nobody!   _____

Scoring

For question #1:
A response: give 15 points = _____
B response: give 7 points = _____
C response: give 1 points = _____

For questions #2—67:
A response: give 5 points = _____
B response: give 3 points = _____
C response: give 1 point = _____

Total of the above points = _____

Interpretation

170—315: PROBABLY Eldic type

92—169: POSSIBLY Eldic type

<92: NOT Eldic type

The Eldic Type

Rocine: "Eldic means 'the potential for looking old and dry'". You absorb and utilize more <u>sodium and chloride</u> than other types. You are among the longest living people on earth.

———

Your skin is thin and tight when young, but may wrinkle with age because of genetics, diet, dehydration, nutritional problems, excessive sunlight exposure, and particularly from excesses of salt and salty fast foods. You need to nutritionally nurture and protect your skin from the sun. The salt shaker is your poison!

▶ *You may look older than you are and have more potential for skin aging than any other type.*

The males usually have larger ears as seen in George Burns and Ross Perot, outstanding examples of your type, while Marco Rubio and Wolf Blitzer are good current examples.

Typically, you are from short to medium-height (with many jockeys and gymnasts); if tall, about 5'8 is your limit. You have less defined muscles and strength than the *myogenic and desmogenic* types, but when healthy you have great endurance strength (Jack LaLayne). You tend to have longer arms and legs, and a shorter trunk.

You may hold fat due to a fatty sub-type or glandular problem. Some females commonly carry an extra 10-20 pounds, but this weight is relatively easily lost. The men are invariably lean and medium-sized, typically looking like Wolf Blitzer, Dustin Hoffman, or Peter Falk.

Like the *desmogenic and nervimotive* types you may erupt with forceful and righteous anger; but generally, you are calm, tranquil, and self-possessed. You are thoughtfully brave and not overtly courageous like the *desmogenic, carbogenic, and nervimotive* types. Many brave women in the armed services are of your type.

———

Physical Similarity to Other Types

The shorter *myogenic* type (Ted Koppel, Bob Costas) looks somewhat similar.

The lean *carbogenic* type (Alec Baldwin, Berndette Peters) is attractive and more social.

The *medeic* type (Mick Jagger, Madonna) is dramatic, intelligent, and usually leaner.

———

Average Height and Weight

> Males: 5'0-5'7 120–170 pounds
> Females: 4'8-5'6 100–160 pounds
> (*Eldics, nervimotives, and some pargenics are the shortest types.*)

———

Eldic Type Description

The type description represents how you appear in everyday society. You may have a sub-type that alters parts of this description.

Think of the celebrity examples as you read the descriptions. You often have a freckled skin with red-brown or darker hair. You are of short to medium-height, never tall, and may have a terse mouth and lips, with larger ears. Note that *eldic* is a common sub-type as seen in Clark Gable; he had the ears but was a *myogenic* type. The males often look wiry. If a bully picks a fight with you he will have a difficult time! You are shapely, often attractive or handsome, and physically, mentally, and ethically strong.

Head — You have a medium-sized, proportioned head, some having a high crown (common with a *myogenic* sub-type).

Hair — Your hair is coarse, dry, strong, and often brunette, black, red or brown. You are rarely balding, usually having a full head of hair throughout life (unless there is a balding sub-type).

Eyes — Sunken eyes with low-set eyebrows slanting towards the nose are common; the eyes appear kind and interested.

Ears — The male ears are usually markedly larger than average: they may flap like Ross Perot's, or be only slightly larger than normal. The ears are un-proportional to other facial aspects and may be odd-shaped (as seen in *neurogenic* men). The female ears are more moderate-sized, sometimes larger with aging.

▶ *In some classic eldics the ears may reach from the eyebrows to below the level of the mouth (as in George Burns)! In other types, large ears represent an eldic sub-type (as in Fred Astaire and Clark Gable).*

Nose — Some have a long thin nose, while others are normal.

Face — Your face sometimes wrinkles from dehydration and aging, which in males may become deep lines and cracks, a classic example being Stanley Holloway who played Liza's father in the film "My Fair Lady". This genetic aspect greatly concerns the ladies who need to protect and nurture their skin!

▶ *There is often a triangular shape to the lower face (like many nervimotives).*

The more the sun abuses your skin, the greater potential for skin aging. You have a long upper jaw, a triangular lower jaw, and a somewhat pointed chin that may be small or moderate-sized.

Mouth and Lips — Your voice is nasal, unique, individual, distinctive, and low-pitched; you have a measured speech, and a talent for talking, public speaking, singing, and readily expressing your truth. Like the ears, the mouth is often an important diagnostic aspect of your type.

▶ *Your mouth is often wide and flat compared to the average person. In many males the lower lip is tight or taunt, and less so in females. The upper lip tends to be thin and firm—the lips may be terse (particularly in males).*

Teeth — Dentition is of high quality, denoting strong calcium metabolism when young. The shape and color of the teeth is normal, but with aging poor nutrition causes yellowing.

Skin —Your skin freckles and tans easily; it is firm, tight, healthy, tough, and leathery. Many fine wrinkles occur with aging that may proceed to creases and a weather–beaten appearance in old age (particularly after many years in the sun). You need daily skin moisteners.

Neck — A small tightly muscled and strong neck is typical; you may undergo skin wrinkling in the neck.

Muscles —You have muscles with endurance potential: newspaper pictures of men and women, running marathons and body-building in their 90's and 100's, are invariably *eldics*.

▶ *I saw a very fit eldic man, age 86, punch out a rude 25year-old bully who was much taller than he.*

Chest — A strong chest, full and wide from side to side is common. You have excellent lung volume and a distinctive speaking or singing voice. The bust comes in all sizes (depending on the sub-type).

Back and Shoulders —The back and shoulders are very strong, muscular and able to carry a heavy load.

Hips and Abdomen — These are normal-sized with easy fat management.

Arms, Legs, Joints — The limbs, normally proportioned, have very flexible and strong joints, hence the Olympic gymnasts and jockeys of your type; with an incorrect diet there is arthritis potential.

* * *

Eldic Personality Traits

If you are this Muscle type many, but not all, of the following characteristics are present—you may have overcome or moderated the negatives, but recognize that you once had several of them.

You may have any of the following traits.

- Ethical and honest
- Dislike wasting time
- Entrepreneur talents
- Appear neutral, indifferent
- Are patriotic and hero-loving
- High self-confidence and self-image
- Are calm, reserved, quiet, in control
- Enjoy hot weather, dislike intense cold
- Very private, restrained, quiet, reserved
- Are inspirational, motivated, reliable, loyal

- Appear composed, whether you are or not
- Would strongly defend honor and promises
- Often attracted to antiquity, tradition, history
- Dislike people who do not follow societal rules
- Peaceful, loving, humorous, law-abiding, fear evil
- Self-activating, build on talents (are often successful)
- Will not abuse a friendship or tolerate over-familiarity
- You believe: "What others think of me is none of my business."
- Are natural athletes, enjoy sports, tramping, etc. (especially males)
- You speak, live and believe your truth (and expect others to do the same); you always do what is right for you!
- Not surprised by anything that happens in life; are born philosophers and able to adjust to life events.

▶ *You will always stand up for any passionate issue, and are often advocates and feminists. You are 'comfortable in your own skin.'*

———

Potential Challenges

You may have evolved from, or not experienced these general faults, so don't dwell on them.

- May be quite vain
- Want to be in control: are rulers
- If betrayed, trouble will come to someone!
- Expect from others what is expected of self: few people can live up to your ideals
- May have some unusual beliefs or attitudes that the average person does not relate to
- Being diplomatic is difficult (yet, then there's Hillary Clinton!); you always speak your truth no matter what the consequences
- Are own worst enemy: you punish yourself for any real or perceived behavioral errors

▶ *If you relate to any of these challenges, doing something to overcome them serves your evolution.*

_____

Eldic Stress Management

You have strong mental stress prevention giving you a good ability not to internalize this stress into your stomach, adrenals, and immune system. Emotional stress prevention is not strong, and any of the above challenges may need reprogramming help. [If needing help managing these stresses, see my prior books.]

_____

Love

You are secretive with your true feelings, but once friendship is given, you are loyal forever. You tend to mate with people of intelligence, creativity, and idealism, particularly the *carbogenic, isogenic, myogenic, and nitropheric* types. Rocine wrote that you are often attracted to the *lipopheric* type.

* * *

Talents and Vocations

Abilities - *Athletics, sports, executive, arts, teaching*

You appreciate art, law, antiquity, the arts, and enjoy work where honor, principle, and honesty is expected. You have a low-boredom threshold, and may work long hours. The type information cannot predict what or who you will become, but you are capable of bringing a creative excellence or brilliance to whatever you do in life.

▶ *I have known or observed you as actors, photographers, singers, musicians, ministers, many entrepreneurs, office managers, school teachers, new age healers, yoga and metaphysical teachers.*

Inabilities – *Diplomacy*

You are not born diplomats! Like Hillary Clinton, Harry Truman and Ross Perot, you are highly testy, and express yourself passionately.

———

Health Problems

If ill, you commonly experience health problems, or diseases in any of the following organs and tissues:

Skin — Is liable to lesions, cancer, and aging.

Liver — Is weak and vulnerable to becoming toxic and underactive.

Lungs — The lungs are vulnerable to disease.

Cardiovascular System — Excess beef and meat eating threatens your heart health; a high cholesterol is common.

Bones and Joints — These tissues are predisposed to arthritis, stones, and degenerative diseases.

Eldic Acid/Alkaline Factor

[See Chapter 3 for details on this subject, along with the common symptoms found with people of different nervous system dominance.]

For your health and healing, the genetics of your autonomic nervous system predispose you to needing a specific ratio of food acidity to alkalinity. You are born with an **intermediate** constitution, requiring a balance between acid and alkaline-ash foods in your diet. (Ash refers to the minerals left in your body after metabolizing foods.

Your autonomic nervous system genetics are intermediate between the *parasympathetic* and *sympathetic* nervous systems, making this acid/alkaline question less important for you compared to the predominantly acid and alkaline types. Construct this approximate ratio of daily food selections:

50% Fruits, salads, vegetables
50% Proteins, carbohydrates

▶ *Approximate your food ratios. On any particular day, it does not matter if one meal is mostly alkaline and another mostly acid—just try to balance it out for the day! If you make a mistake, try again tomorrow. It is a subjective call that you make; what you do over time makes the difference in your health.*

The Eldic Spiritual Factor

Skip this paragraph if uninterested in a philosophical perspective on your type!

▶ *Rocine: "The soul chooses the body type."*

If as souls, we choose the brain and body type to spend a lifetime in, it could be to learn certain spiritual lessons related to perfecting ourselves, and our humanity, in God's eyes. What lessons does the type bring you? Only you can really decide what those lessons are.

You know things about yourself that Victor Rocine could never get from his research subjects when he first wrote about types. So search your mind for the answers.

Each discrete type has challenges of life lessons, spiritual goals, etc., and some of yours may be:

Faith — Many of you have highly developed faith in something, whether orthodox, metaphysical, or unorthodox.

High Expectations — Accept that others are not like you!

Undiplomatic — You express unadulterated truth (and need to accept that diplomacy is necessary in social interaction).

Controlling — Being overly-strict and controlling of people in your life is a common problem; relax and your loved ones, friends and employees will appreciate you more.

Overly Idealistic — Are highly idealistic; be more accepting of those not sharing your dreams and try to match your goals with what is realistic!

———

An Eldic Story...

Ruth, age 28, suffered from fatigue, back pain, mental stress, and headaches. Examination showed excessive junk foods in her diet, her fears and apathy probably being diet-related. She did emotional releasing, and stopped eating salted foods: salt, catsup, sauerkraut, preserved luncheon meats, and frozen vegetables.

To help normalize her calcium metabolism, she needed healthy sodium foods daily: kelp, olives, cheddar cheese, scallops, cottage cheese, lobster, Swiss chard, beets, and buttermilk. Ruth made the needed changes and her symptoms quickly resolved.

———

Eldic Type Mineral Needs

Apply this mineral data to the diet following the Muscle type descriptions.

Excessive Foods:

- *Sodium, Chlorine (salt, junk foods)*
- *Nitrogen (beef)*

Deficient Foods:

- *Sodium, Chlorine (non-junk)*
- *Potassium*
- *Calcium*
- *Nitrogen (non-beef, vegetable)*

These deficient nutrients are common deficiencies in your type, and predispose you to ill-health.
If ill, be sure to use these lists with your <u>daily</u> food intake.
If not ill, eat from the foods lists 3-4 times <u>weekly</u>.
All food lists are in descending order of concentration and value to you; choose servings of foods in the upper half of each list first!
One serving is 1/2 cup.

Eldic Excessive F oods -

Sodium and Chlorine foods are excessive in your tissues, if ill or diseased; to preserve your health and weight control avoid junk foods, and fulfill these nutrient needs from the food lists (without using the salt shaker).

▶ *Rocine: "Salt, meat eating, especially beef is a major cause of your health problems."*

Nitrogen from red meat is excessive in your diet (if eaten more than 1-2 times monthly).

———

Deficient Foods -

In illness or disease, it is important to correct these mineral deficiencies.

Sodium, Chlorine foods (unsalted) in moderation help your healing; they need replenishing daily in food form.

Potassium is deficient in your type. It is concentrated in and vital to the health of your muscles, heart, brain, and all cells. If ill or diseased, potassium foods and supplements are a significant healing factor.

Calcium is often deficient in your type. It is highly concentrated in bones, joints, muscles, nerves, heart, teeth, and gums; if you have an illness or disease in any of these tissues calcium foods and supplements may be a significant healing factor.

Nitrogen from vegetable and non-red meat sources is deficient (see above notes).

▶ *Even though you might like flesh, your nervous system genetics make you a weak carnivore—your health improves with less flesh intake.*

———

Minimize

Excessive Mineral Foods

Sodium, Chlorine (salted, junk):
0-1 *times/week*

Table salt, all fast foods, packaged foods, canned and frozen foods, soy sauce, all preserved meats (cured, smoked, canned and luncheon meats), sauces (barbecue, catsup, etc.), dill pickles, sauer-kraut, bouillon cubes, peanut butter, potato chips, etc., salted nuts, crackers, canned or packaged soups, processed cheeses, commercial salad dressings, meat tenderizers.

Note: If you must eat anything on the above list, keep it down to ½ cup, once weekly!

Nitrogen (beef): 0-2 *times/month only*

Beef and red meats
Note — Be sure to minimize all caffeine, tea, coffee that dehydrate you, and contribute to skin drying and aging.

Note – *The following recommendations are for the generic type. Additionally, you may need from a holistic healer or nutritionist something more specific for your individuality.*

Eat

Deficient Foods

Potassium: *1-2 servings/day*

Banana, tomatoes, green vegetables, okra, dairy foods, halibut, winter squash, Swiss and cheddar cheese, prunes, sweet potatoes, beet greens, corn.

Sodium, Chlorine (non-junk):
   2-4 servings/week

Kelp, fish, milk, goat (brown or white) cheese and milk, olives, cottage cheese, gizzard, lentils, raw cabbage, almonds, Swiss chard, beet greens, buttermilk, celery, spinach, oysters, chicken.

Calcium: *1-2 servings/day*

Dulse, blackstrap molasses, rice bran, Swiss cheese; cabbage, turnip, green vegetable and citrus fruits (and their juices); almonds, brewer's yeast, parsley, whole wheat, sunflower and sesame seeds, raisins, corn tortilla, dandelion green.

Nitrogen (non-beef, vegetable):

Legumes, peas, beans, black-eyed peas, seeds, nuts, pasta, spirulina, soy (tofu) — as desired
Eggs, poultry, fish — 3-4 times/week

Note: Eat any healthy foods you desire, but be sure to include the type foods in your daily choices.

Eldic Nutritional Supplements

- **Multi-Vitamins** —
  [Take all supplements with food]
  2 capsules/day

- **Calcium** —
  600 mg/twice daily

- **Potassium** —
  About 200 mg/day with food
  [Or take a multi-vitamin-mineral
  containing the above nutrients.]

- **Herbs** —
  Brain detox – Gingko or Gotu Kola
  Organ detox – White Willow or
  Chickweed
  (Take one capsule, twice daily, for one
  month; then one, three times weekly.)

- **Lecithin** —
  About 1,300 mg/three times weekly

- **Evening Primrose or Flaxseed Oil**
  Take one soft-gel daily with food.

Note: Be sure to take these supplements if you
have ill-health. If in good health, take them at
least 3-4 days weekly.

Important Eldic Health Concerns

Any instinctive carnivorous cravings are normal and healthy for you, as long as you do not overdo it! You need the *Muscle* type food guide, with less flesh: eat about four vegetarian days and three flesh days/week.

You need potassium foods, green salads and vegetables, and some flesh in your diet; you are *not* born to be pure vegetarians although some of you may choose to be; if so, pay particular attention to your daily protein intake with a protein drink (about 30-35 gm/day).

▶ *Rocine: "You need about ten times more potassium foods than sodium and chlorine foods in your diet. You need some food sodium, but not salted foods!"*

You often have food allergies and sensitivities to certain grains, fruits, alcohol, and sugar. Identify them and avoid those foods! Dairy allergy is common.

<u>*Eldic Food Guide*</u>

Aim for -
50% Proteins, complex carbohydrates
50% Fruits, salads, vegetables
and
50% Raw food diet
50% Cooked foods

<u>Stay hydrated (8 plus glasses daily)</u>
<u>Dump the salt shaker!</u>
Take the recommended supplements.

Eldic Weight Loss

Losing weight is relatively easy and depends upon you following the type instructions summarized in this section:

- *Stop* eating salt and salted foods!
- *Protein* drink daily, have about 25-30 grams
- *Eat* your body type deficient mineral foods daily
- *Follow* your *Eldic Guide (as above)*
- *Exercise*: your body type requires moderate to intense daily exercise

- *Simple sugars:* stop all white table sugar and high-fructose corn syrup and drinks containing these sugars
- *Mental balance and positive thinking:* you may be mentally stressed by everyday life, which causes adrenal hypoglycemia, low blood sugar; you need to take these supplements: *calcium/magnesium,* two capsules, twice daily with food; and *chamomile,* two capsules with food
- *Hypoglycemia:* this hormonal imbalance stops fat loss, and usually initiates more fat production, so it is vital to deal with this problem: take *pantothenic acid,* 500 mg/twice daily with food
- *Calories:* As with any dietary approach, calories in, must be *less than* calories out! Most markets sell a calorie booklet; make notes of your daily intake, and in most instances keep it under about 1500 calories/day

———

Muscle Types
General Food Guide

(Carnivores)

Important Note

————

The Food Guide addresses the <u>Acid-Alkaline</u> aspect of your food intake, along with the <u>Type Mineral</u> factor presented throughout this book. It does <u>not</u> necessarily address calories or other dietary factors that may be pertinent to your personal health needs whether medical or appropriate for some other dietary need. So use your common sense and just include the factors described here with whatever healthy dietary choices you usually make.

For other nutrient information, consult with nutritional books or with holistic nutritional doctors. I particularly recommend the advice of Andrew Weil, M.D.

————

Muscle Types
General Food Guide

(Not for the Nitropheric Type)

This chapter presents a general Food Guide, upon which you superimpose the nutritional information from your type chapter. As a Muscle body type your genetics require flesh foods.

Meat/Flesh Intake

Most muscle types should limit red meat to once or less weekly, while eggs, lamb, fish, or poultry are excellent in moderation. If ill or diseased, be sure to eat daily, one or two servings from each *deficient minerals* list. If not ill, eat them at least three times weekly for health maintenance. If this diet is similar to your present diet, but healing is sluggish, then:

- Decrease your carbohydrate and protein intake by about one-third
- Increase your fruit, salad, and vegetable intake by about one-third
- Consult with a holistic doctor, preferably one versed in nutritional and emotional evaluation

-----

Over-Acid or Over-Alkaline?

Just as a log of wood burned in your fireplace leaves a mineral-ash, food ash refers to the minerals remaining after metabolizing foods in your tissues:

- Fruits, vegetables **alkalinize** tissues
- Proteins, carbohydrates **acidify** tissues

Usually You Are Over-Acid Due To:

- Excessive intake of dairy foods
- Excessive intake of proteins and carbohydrates
- Deficient intake of fruits, salads and vegetables
- Accumulated metabolic waste-acids (from years of eating excessive acid-ash foods, meats and carbohydrates, and from lack of exercise)
- You need to estimate the ratio of foods eaten. Generally, eat the following *approximate* ratios for your health:

50% **<u>Alkaline-ash</u>** foods *(fruits, salads, vegetables)*

50% **<u>Acid-ash</u>** foods *(complex carbo-hydrates like starches, grains, cereals, breads, flour products; and proteins)*

Approximate your food ratios. On any particular day, it does not matter if one meal is mostly alkaline, and another mostly acid—just try to balance it out for the day! If you get it wrong, try again tomorrow. It is a subjective call that you make, and it is what you do over weeks, months, or years that make the difference—not on any one or two days.

―――――

Note - If Vegetarian

As a general indication, if you follow a vegetarian diet substitute vegetable sources of protein for the any flesh in the food guide. Note that contrary to most alkaline-ash vegetarian diets you need something different:

*You need an **acid-ash** vegetarian diet high in complex carbohydrates and vegetable proteins.*

Because of your high need for protein, you usually require a vegetable powdered protein supplement in juice (about 25-30 grams daily).

―――――

Important

- Minimize white sugar and alcohol intake.
- If desired, interchange lunches for dinners.

- Never eat foods you are allergic to, no matter what I recommend; if allergic, or suspect a food allergy, eliminate it and substitute from your type mineral lists.
- Eat the right foods 80-90% of the time and the Food Guide will work for you; unlike some types you do not have to live out of a health food store (although such foods are healthier for you).

▶ *Omit eating the excessive minerals in your type chapter, and be sure to eat one or two servings from the deficient list daily.*

Finally, in addition to your body type needs, other holistic healing matters also need your attention. I strongly suggest that you refer to my web site and earlier books for that information: *DrStenbeck.net*

_____

Acid/Alkaline Genetics Chart

The following chart reflects each Muscle Type and its acid or alkaline-ash food needs. These ratios change if you are unhealthy or over age 45-50. Refer back to your body type and review the *Acid/alkaline* instructions.

_____

Acid/Alkaline Genetics, Dietary-Ash, and Raw Food Needs

This chart shows the Rocine types, their acid or alkaline food needs, and the percentage of raw foods needed for your health and healing.

- Apply your Type Minerals to the Food Guide

Type	Acid/Alkaline Genetics	% Food-Ash Needed	% Raw Food Needed
Calciferic	Alkaline	70% acid	30
Carbogenic	Alkaline	50-50	50
Desmogenic	Alkaline	70% acid	50
Eldic	Intermediate	50-50	50
Medeic	Intermediate	50-50	50
Myogenic	Intermediate	50-50	50
Nervimotive	Alkaline	70% acid	50
Nitropheric	Acid	70% alkaline	70
Pallinomic	Alkaline	50-50	30

The above percentages vary depending on aging and the health of individual types.

Muscle Types / Food Guide
<u>*Breakfast*</u>

[Superimpose the nutritional information from your

EGGS (1-2) with lettuce, tomato, or salad,   whole grain toast; (add bacon or sausage 1-3 times weekly if desired)
— 2-4 times/week; or*

*FRUIT fresh salad, and protein (yogurt, milk, cheeses, seeds, nuts)
—1-3 times/week; or*

*CEREALS, with fruit, seeds, nuts
—2-5 times/week; or*

*OTHER choices
— 0-1 times weekly*

<u>*Daily liquids:*</u>
Pure water, citrus, vegetable juices, soups, other — as desired
Coffee, teas —0-2 cups

[Include selections from your type mineral needs everyday.]

Muscle Types / Food Guide

Lunch

SALADS, *mixed green, protein (poultry, fish, egg, cheese, seeds or nuts, etc.), whole grain breads*
[Dressing: olive oil/vinegar; low-fat, low-cal dressings]
— 2-4 times/week; or

SANDWICH, whole grains with a protein (cheese, tuna, ham, etc.); and salad and/or vegetables
— 1-4 times/week; or

POULTRY OR FISH 3-6 oz., *with a mixed green salad and/or vegetables*
—1-3 times/week; or

OTHER *choices (with salad or vegetables)*
—1-2 times/week

[Other oils permitted, soybean oil is a common allergen; minimize commercial dressings. Include two or more selections from your type food lists in your daily food intake. For snacks, eat fruit or vegetables with seeds/nuts.]

Muscle Types / Food Guide
<u>Dinner</u>

POULTRY OR FISH *(4-6 oz.), with salad and/ or vegetables*
—2-4 times/week; or

PASTA *with protein (chicken, etc.) with salad and/ or vegetables*
— 2-4 times/week; or

VEGETARIAN *meal with salad and/ or vegetables*
—1-3 times/week; or

LEAN BEEF *(4-6 oz.) with salad and/ or vegetables*
— 0-1 times/week

OTHER *choices with salad and/ or vegetables*
— 0-1 times/week

<u>*Desserts:*</u>
Fruits, fresh — as desired
Low-sugar, healthy desserts
— 0-3 times/wk

Food Guide Notes

Steamed Vegetables —

Minerals are lost in the boiling of vegetables; steaming or wok cooking is best.

Food Combinations —

If you have a weak digestive system then eating proteins at the same meal with starches often results in indigestion, gas, or constipation.

Periodic Detox —

You tend to over-indulge in acid-ash foods (proteins and carbohydrates), and often need occasional elimination diets for tissue waste-acid removal. Have a holistic doctor or nutritionist supervise such detox (where you have an alkaline-ash diet along with protein supplementation).

Minimize —

- Fatty foods
- Commercial salad dressings
- Beef, red meats, processed meats
- Coffee, white sugar, corn syrup, alcohol

Vegetarian Proteins —

You require a carnivorous diet. An exception is the *nitropheric* type who functions best with a *vegetarian* diet. The other muscle types are born to be carnivores. It is very difficult for the other muscle types to be pure vegetarians because of their strong intuitive cravings for fish, poultry, meat, or eggs. If you are vegetarian, then because of your high needs for amino acids and acid-ash foods, you should take a protein supplement of 30-40 grams/day (powdered protein in juice).

Healthy Weight —

Several of you gain weight as the ravages of age, lack of exercise and dietary excesses take their toll. By eating according to your body type, you should naturally lose excess weight. Each type also has a few individual factors that only apply to them!

You have a good ability to lose weight by following the Food Guide instructions. The most common problem I find with your weight-control is liver and kidney irritation due to food allergies, which results in extra pounds. The key is to eat non-allergic foods.

If drinking more than 3-4 cups daily of coffee or tea, you may have a hypoglycemic problem (low blood sugar), which contributes to making fat, ill-health, and delayed healing. (Refer to the earlier books for help with this healing.)

———

Appendix

Brief Extracts from
"The 22 Unique Body Types"

————

Appendix A

Types
(Brief extract)

Type comes from 'typus' meaning an image or impression, the study of types being called typology.

▶ *Rocine: "A combination of mental and structural features is consistently found in people of the same type."*

Rocine wrote that all types are a mixture of positive and negative qualities. He based his work on the biochemical individuality of our *mineral* absorption and utilization. Of course, all minerals are absorbed, but he postulated that different types of people *selectively* absorb certain minerals, to a greater or lesser extent, requiring specific mineral foods for their enhanced health and healing. This is the basis of his types.

▶ *The type information cannot predict what or who you will become, or how successful or not, but your type is capable of bringing a creative excellence to whatever you do in life. If your type has negative qualities that you disagree with, remember that they are only tendencies and may or may not manifest in you.*

This book enlarges on Rocine's premise (early 1900's), integrated with the later research of Herbert Sheldon, M.D., Ph.D., at Harvard University (1930's), along with my fifty years of observations and experience with this subject.

Comparing your shared physical (and sometimes psychological) descriptions with the Celebrity Lists further assists the identification of your type. It is not that you will look exactly like, or be a twin to, any particular celebrity. Look closely at a celebrity's features: face, profile, height, weight, head, etc. If you know something about their talents, beliefs, success and failure spheres, health and weight challenges, attitudes and behaviors, etc., then you get clues as to what your type may be.

———

Understanding Types and Sub-Types

Each of us has a clearly discernible dominant type. Visualize the celebrity examples from movies, politics, sports, the arts and public life, and try to identify with their physical features. Look for similar features, remembering that you will not recognize all attributes in yourself. You are not looking for your twin!

The sub-type issue is the main reason people of the same major type can look so different. Remember that a type description does not characterize you exactly, but depicts your individual variant of a type.

▶ *The type questionnaire pinpoints the major features of that type: if the celebrity examples are unhelpful, you may be an unusual variant (in which case ignore the celebrity issue and give yourself 7 points on Question 1).*

Minerals
(Brief extract)

Minerals are essential life nutrients that accelerate enzyme and chemical reactions and provide a basis for your body typing. Although found in all tissues, different minerals tend to be concentrated in certain organs, their presence or absence contributing to the healing of such tissues; e.g., zinc accelerates prostate healing; calcium and manganese promote bone, joint and connective tissue healing.

Specific foods nurture each type, some people needing meats for their health others needing a vegetarian diet. A high potassium diet nurtures one person, while another needs high sulfur, calcium, zinc, or another mineral.

Mineral Digestion and Absorption

Compared to vitamins, minerals are *difficult* to digest, absorb, and utilize. In people with strong digestive systems, this aspect may not be important. The following factors should be in place for optimal mineral metabolism:

1. Stomach Hydrochloric Acid Production
2. Parathyroid Hormone Balance
3. Organ Toxic Metal and Chemical Removal
   [See details in The 22 Unique Body Types.*]*

Total Body Healing

Note that from a holistic healing perspective, in addition to minerals and type information, address these healing factors:

Nutrient Balance
Mental Balance
Emotional Balance
Spiritual Balance
Detoxifying Integrity

The above factors are all important to your total healing especially if you are interested in self-healing (see my earlier books).

Appendix B

Researchers
(Brief extract)

The predominant workers in this area of human individuality from around 1880's to the 1960's are Herbert Sheldon, M.D., Ph.D., Roger Williams, Ph.D., and Victor Rocine, D.Sc.

Much information on Sheldon's research exists on-line and in medical psychology libraries; for interested readers there are other lines of research published in the last century. This present book is primarily about Rocine's body types.

Herbert Sheldon M.D., Ph.D.

In contrast to Rocine, Sheldon at Harvard University in the 1930's was trained in the scientific method and did painstaking research and publishing on human individuality. In comparing his findings with Rocine's work, a direct putative correlation is visible.

Roger J. Williams, Ph.D.

Another significant researcher in human individuality is the renowned scientist and

biochemist, Roger J. Williams. He demon-
strated that different people have varying
levels of nutrients, enzymes, and other
metabolic chemicals in their bloodstreams.

▶ *Williams's research firmly expands on the*
premise of individual nutritional needs in human
beings. If interested in his research, I highly
recommend his book Biochemial Individuality.

Victor Rocine, D.Sc.

Note that when a negative feature is
indicated, say neurotic tendencies, all members
of the type are <u>not</u> that way; it is a type tendency
reported by Rocine.

Rocine studied type-related diseases finding
links between mineral and dietary factors with
individual types and their diseases. In each
body type, one or more dominant minerals are
preferentially absorbed and utilized over other
minerals.

He recognized discrete body types from their
physical appearance finding genetically based
mineral dominance to be the determining feature.
He also correlated their physical features with
psychological characteristics.

———

Appendix C

Genetics, Types, and Diet
(Brief extract)

This section deals with how nervous system genetics helps determine your eating choices for health: you are either born to be a predominant meat eater, a partial or complete vegetarian, or something between the two. The genetic factor determining this dietary aspect is the *sympathetic and parasympathetic* components of your central nervous system. This represents a basic factor in eating for health.

This chapter helps you understand your dietary inheritance, although instinctively, you may already have arrived there!

- If born **sympathetic** dominant you are *genetically acid*, desiring a predominantly *vegetarian* diet for your health (about 70% fruit, salad, vegetables to 30% proteins and carbohydrates).

- If born **parasympathetic** dominant you are *genetically alkaline*, desiring a predominantly *carnivorous* diet for your health (70% proteins, carbohydrates). You rarely choose vegetarianism because of the difficulty in satisfying your protein needs without meats.

- If born *intermediate* dominant you may eat food groups with little concern for the acid/alkaline factor. However, after age 40, you need a semi-vegetarian diet for healthy eating.

———

Chart of Relative Nervous System Dominance

In the following Chart, if you relate to many of the symptoms on one side you probably have that nervous system dominance; relating to both sides indicates *Intermediate* dominance.

If Vegetarian (Over-acid)
Eat 70% fruits, salads, vegetables
And 30% proteins, carbohydrates

If Carnivore (Over-alkaline)
Eat 70% proteins, carbohydrates
And 30% fruits, salads, vegetables

If Intermediate
Eat 50:50 of acid and alkaline-ash foods

Make an *approximate* estimate of your daily acid and alkaline food intake (such ratios varying from type to type).

———

Symptoms of Relative Genetic Dominance

Vegetarians (Over-acid)	Carnivores (Over-alkaline)
Sympathetic Dominance	Parasympathetic Dominance
little or no flesh desire	desire flesh
easily constipated	rarely constipated
slow digestion	fast digestion
easily dehydrated	not dehydrated
strong thirst	low thirst
pale face	flushed face
high pulse after food	slow pulse after food
easy gag reflex	slow gag reflex
cool dry skin	moist warm skin
nervous stomach	calm stomach
little eyelid blinking	much blinking
nervous tendency	mostly calm
slower healing	faster healing
low oxygen-uptake	good oxygen-uptake
easily breathless	seldom breathless
insomnia common	sleep easier
few muscle cramps	some night cramps
calcium deposits rare	get calcium deposits

Appendix D

Help Identifying your Body Type with Dr. Stenbeck

If you desire help in identifying your body type, follow these instructions, and answer the questionnaire. For further information and fees, send me an email from page one of the website:

DrStenbeck.net

First name: _____

Country of birth: _____

Upload photos and send to the above website:

- Head and shoulders: front and side views

- Full body: front and side views

- Also 1-2 teenage views

- If possible, casual photos of mother, father, siblings

MY TYPE CLASS MAY BE: _____

    (Thin, Muscle, or Fat)

AGE   -   _____

HEIGHT   -   _____ feet/inches

MY WEIGHT -   _____ pounds

- Heaviest at age: _____

- Lightest as adult: _____

- Estimate age 15: _____

VISION - Excellent   Average   Poor:

HAIR -   Natural color: _____

- Thin/thick? _____

- balding? _____

SKIN - Quality: _____

- History of acne, boils, other:

_____

_____

TEETH -   Strong   Weak   Dentures

- Cavity history: Many   Moderate   Few

MUSCLES   -   Strong   Average   Weak

Sports played _____

JOINTS -   Strong   Average   Weak

HEALTH - Childhood diseases?

_____

_____

- Adult diseases?

_____

AVERAGE DIET

- Beef _____ (times/week)

- Poultry _____ (times/week)

- Fish _____ (times/week)

- Eggs _____ (times/week)

- Water _____ (glasses/day):

- Vegetarian? Vegan? _____

- Other? _____

- Did your childhood diet differ? _____

The above will help me know who you are! I will send you a follow-up questionnaire for further help in identifying your body type.

Appendix E

On-line Health Consultation with Dr. Stenbeck

For further information, or to comment on this book, or to receive a response on any health issue from a holistic viewpoint, send an email inquiry from page one of my website:

DrStenbeck.net

Following that, I will suggest further healing needs, which we may pursue with an on-line consult.

———

Appendix F

Notes

See my book *The 22 Unique Body Types,* available at the usual online source, for further information and details on all of the 22 Types. The Appendix in that book also has more information about:

- *Mineral Functions and Food Sources*

- *Further Reading*

_____

www.ingramcontent.com/pod-product-compliance
Lightning Source LLC
Chambersburg PA
CBHW062102280526
45788CB00003B/1319